YOUR GUIDE TO ASSISTED LIVING IN ARIZONA

YOUR GUIDE TO ASSISTED LIVING IN ARIZONA

What You Should Know before Placing Your Loved One

By Russell and Tammy Burns

ISBN: 978-0-557-43305-6

CONTENTS

Preface

This book is the result of our learning the assisted living industry from the inside out. At the time of writing we have been caring for people for five years. During those five years we have learned our role in caregiving and have also seen the frustrations families experience as they attempt to navigate the long-term care system. With this book, we wish to provide a tool for our own families and for others who will be facing the many decisions related to long-term care in the very near future.

We have chosen to write from *us* to *you*. We will be assuming that you are the one pursuing long-term care options for *your loved one* or for *Mom* or *Dad, Grandpa, Aunt Sally, etc.* and will use those terms interchangeably with *resident*.

We also are writing from the point of view of assisted-living home care. Our greatest experience caring for people is in a ten-bed home environment, although we interact regularly with larger facilities and with people in their own homes. We believe that for the majority of those requiring assistance, the assisted-living home is by far the best alternative, and this book will primarily deal with that context. But there are times when a larger center is advantageous. Some of these advantages are listed here.

- **Transportation:** Large centers generally provide a schedule of regular outings to various shopping locations around town (Kmart, Wal-Mart, grocery stores, shopping malls) in addition to individual appointments. These may or may not be charged separately.
- **Activities:** Most large centers have an extensive activity program. If this is of interest to you, be sure to visit during those activities and see who participates and if it is indeed what you have in mind.
- **Dining:** Generally restaurant-style dining is available with various selections, as opposed to homestyle cooking where everyone eats basically the same menu.
- **Community:** In a larger center there is a larger community and therefore a greater likelihood that you will find compatible people to relate to.
- **In-house services:** Often the larger center will have an onsite hair salon, gift shop, rehab or exercise facility, and other services that might be of interest to you.
- **Medical services:** If you require skilled nursing services on an ongoing basis, larger skilled nursing centers may be your only option. This may vary, as many conditions can be treated in the smaller home setting through home health agencies. Discuss this with the home if you would prefer a home atmosphere, and they can tell you exactly what they can and cannot do.

We want this guide to be a simple and practical tool for you to gain some understanding of the major issues you will be facing, so we have intentionally tried to reduce the clutter of excessive information within the primary text. At the end of the book are appendices containing useful forms, checklists, and instructions for navigating through various aspects of the healthcare system in Arizona. We are also maintaining new and current information and FAQs on our website at www .arizonahomestead.com for you to access at any time.

Introduction

THE NEED FOR THIS BOOK

This guidebook is a must-have for anyone approaching the season of overseeing a loved one's needs. It was written *with you in mind*. You might be a doctor or an RN, a son or daughter, or a neighbor. You might be anyone who is or knows a person approaching the need for some form of long-term care. Hopefully, you are in a position of planning ahead for what may be coming down the road. *Do not wait* until you find yourself needing long-term care for a loved one. Research the options early and know what you will be facing should the need arise.

This guide is designed to empower you, the consumer in the long-term care system, so that you can make informed decisions and at the same time raise the standard of adult assisted living in our community. As you, the average citizen, are informed and educated, the industry will automatically rise up to meet the higher demand. This is our desire: the highest standard of care for those requiring it and your confidence as you place them. By understanding your options, you will be able to make the best decisions in highly stressful situations.

> **Our purpose is to help you understand the system and your role in it, to define reasonable expectations, and to give you the tools you need to secure the best care.**

THE BABY BOOMERS

They're coming—it's no secret! The baby boomers are rounding the final curve of life and entering into that blessed season called retirement and senior citizenship. In 2006 the first baby boomer turned sixty, officially cracking open the floodgates. As with every season of the life of this generation, the entire nation will shift in order to meet their demands. They needed diapers and baby food in the 1940s and 1950s and fast food in the 1950s and 1960s. They participated in the housing boom in the 1970s and the credit craze in the 1980s and 1990s. Now they're ushering their kids out into the world and beginning to enjoy the empty nest.

Close on the horizon comes the season of Medicare, Social Security, and the ever-looming long-term care. Analysts have talked about this coming event for years. Will Medicare and Social Security hold up? We will soon see.

What will happen, regardless, is that we will have a huge population requiring all kinds of medical and daily-living assistance. It will fall, in most cases, to their children to walk down this road with them. We have walked it with various people and are convinced a guidebook like this will be not merely helpful but indispensable in the quest for care for Mom and Dad, not just adequately but superbly.

THE NATURE OF THE TASK

The need for this book arises from a number of other realities in our world as well. First, almost all of us, finding ourselves in the position of securing long-term care for a loved one, are novices. Rarely do we do this for more than a few people in our lifetime—our parents, maybe an aunt or uncle, a grandparent, or a close friend. Not only do we generally have just a few people in our lives in this season of life, but not all of them will require long-term care. The majority of us will find ourselves caring for just one or two folks with these needs. When we start, we're uneducated, and when we finish, we may understand the system better than we'd like to, but most likely we will not need to go through it again.

SYSTEM BREAKDOWN

In light of the above, the consumer (that's you) is largely at the mercy of the system, and that's a very scary place to be. Our system is not designed to be helpful. Most people you talk to will know their own area of expertise and little else.

Furthermore, nearly every agency out there, regardless of what they tell you, represents someone who is making money by way of your loved one's care, and they will usually lead you into the arena that pays them the best. Most of the time they mean well, but it's big business, and unfortunately, too often it is designed with profits as the goal, not the best care for your loved one.

> **Whether good or bad, the system is all we have. We hope to guide you step by step through it, taking out some of the mystery and positioning you to make the best decisions regarding the care of your loved one.**

If you have ever participated in the healthcare system, whether through a brief stay in the hospital or an extended illness involving many practitioners, you know that the system is lacking at best. Of course, within the system there are those who genuinely care and who are acutely interested in you and in your loved one's well-being. But the reality is that the system is filled with rules and regulations designed ostensibly to protect you but in fact result from endless lawsuits. The majority of rules are designed to protect the institutions. So we are left with a confusing web of bureaucracy through which we must navigate in order to secure the assistance we need.

The healthcare system is fragmented, with many individual entities providing specific services and under strict legal obligations to protect privacy. This inhibits the flow of communication from one branch of the system to another and creates huge obstacles in the ability of the system to educate and support and to provide continuity of care.

As we have counseled many people through the process of caring for a loved one in the long-term-care system, we have found a great many repeating scenarios. We will share fictional scenarios based on real-life experiences throughout the book so that you may find stories similar to yours.

CHAPTER 1

Be Proactive: Make a Plan Before the Need Arises

Grace's Story

It was a warm day in June when Grace woke up early in the morning in her own bedroom in the eastern suburbs of Tucson. At 88, she had always been healthy and proud of her ability to care for herself and not burden her family. She saw her doctor once or twice a year and took only a pill for her thyroid and a multivitamin each day. Her father had lived to be 97 and her mother 102. Grace had a number of good years left ahead of her, and she took good care of herself so that she could enjoy them independently. Her husband had passed away two years earlier. She missed him, but she kept herself busy and believed that she still had a purpose on earth.

As she sat up to head to the bathroom, she felt a bit dizzy. She had been feeling a little weak and under the weather the past couple of days and thought maybe she had a touch of something going around. Maybe she just needed to drink more water, she thought. That was probably it. She would make that a point, but then, of course, there were the endless trips to the bathroom that came with that, which seemed to be increasing these days and becoming more urgent, like now.

Grace stood up a little before she should have, and her legs just seemed to give out from underneath her. She stumbled to catch her balance, but to no avail. She crashed to the floor, toppling over a TV tray containing last night's dishes on her way down. Moments later, she opened her eyes. She wasn't sure if she had passed out and was waking up or if she had just fallen. She looked around and tried to move. That's when she became aware of an excruciating pain on her left side. She could not move without pain shooting everywhere and nearly causing her to go unconscious.

She felt for her Life Alert button, but it wasn't there. She had taken it off last night in the shower and had forgotten to put it back on. This was very uncharacteristic of her. Everything seemed to spin inside her head from the pain and the confusion about what she should do. She tried calling out for help, but because she lived in a single-family house, she really didn't expect anyone to hear her. There was no phone within reach, and besides, her family had just left for a weekend vacation. She lay there in shock and pain, unsure of what to do next. She felt very frightened.

She wasn't sure how much time had passed when she woke up in the hospital. Her neighbor, Lois, was standing by her bed. Lois explained that she had come by that afternoon with some nut bread she had made, and when Grace didn't answer the door, she suspected something might be wrong. She went home and tried to call, but no one answered. She had tried to come into the house, but it was all locked up, so she took a risk and called 911. The paramedics had found Grace unconscious on the floor and brought her to the emergency room. But Grace had no idea who Lois was or why she might have found her on the floor. She tried to get up, but she was hooked up to all kinds of machines. She asked for her husband and demanded that he be notified right away. Lois explained to the doctor that this was not like Grace. She was almost never confused.

When asked about a power of attorney or anyone who might be designated to make decisions on Grace's behalf, Lois was unable to answer. Lois explained that Grace's daughter was out of town on vacation. She had called her and was waiting to hear back. Meanwhile, Grace was explaining that her daughter would be of no use in this situation because she was only a child. She insisted that they ought to contact her husband.

Suddenly, Lois's cell phone rang. It was Grace's daughter. Lois explained the situation to her, and she said they would come right away, but it would probably be a day before they could make it back. She asked to talk to the medical team at the hospital but was told that they could not share anything about the patient's condition because they had no written or verbal permission to do so.

This story is all too typical. Many of Grace's problems could have been avoided, but they also could have been much more complicated. This story brings up many issues that people may be unaware of, from health risks to interfacing with the medical system to the question of who will make decisions for Grace if she doesn't recover her faculties.

Grace suffered from a urinary tract infection (UTI) that had made her weak and unable to get to the bathroom in time. A UTI can come on quickly and make a perfectly sane person crazy almost overnight. It also causes weakness and a need to urinate frequently. In the elderly, it is not always accompanied by discomfort.

Because Grace was the picture of health, she hadn't made plans yet for someone to have her medical power of attorney in the event that she should become unable to make decisions herself. Grace was at the mercy of the system, which is designed to make money and protect itself from lawsuits first, and then to do its best for the patient second.

In Grace's case, the doctors ran tests, discovered the UTI, and put her on antibiotics. The fall had caused a broken left hip that would require surgery. By the time the family arrived the following morning, Grace was back to her sharp self and was able to give consent for the family to make decisions on her behalf. Suddenly the family was placed in the overwhelming position of taking care of Mom, who would very likely not be able to return home and live alone again.

OBTAIN NECESSARY DOCUMENTS EARLY

This story is a classic example of the need for everyone to have some plan or to be thinking about long-term care solutions for their loved ones much earlier than may seem necessary. In Grace's case, the need was sudden and obvious. Often it is not so clear. We cannot stress enough the importance of establishing your plans and legal authority to represent your loved one as early as possible.

> **Discussing these matters before any signs of decline present themselves can radically reduce conflict. Both parties can plan for the inevitable without having the inevitable bearing down on them.**

Medical and Financial Powers of Attorney

It's never too early for emergency planning, but it can quickly become too late. Planning can be further complicated when a parent feels threatened by their children moving into a parenting role. Discussing these things long before any signs of decline present themselves can radically reduce this conflict, as both parties can plan for the inevitable without having to say that the inevitable is upon them. Furthermore, planning ahead for a parent's long-term care needs will save hundreds and maybe thousands of dollars, not to mention endless stress, time, and hassle.

Jim's Story

Jim, eighty-seven, had lived alone in his home in Scottsdale ever since his wife, Margaret, passed away. She had had a very slow-progressing form of cancer, and Jim had cared for her meticulously during the last five years of her life. They had hired a housekeeper some ten years before her passing, and this housekeeper, Patricia, had gradually become somewhat of a caregiver, assisting Jim in the care of his wife. Patricia was a very hard worker and was extremely devoted to Margaret and Jim.

Jim had very high standards and an extremely high level of compassion. When Margaret died, Jim felt that it made sense to have Patricia move in and become a full-time house-keeper/caregiver for him, as there were many things he was beginning to need assistance with, and he didn't think he should be home alone. He had two children: a daughter, Monica, in Flagstaff, and a son, Mike, in Florida. Although they called and visited from time to time, they never really interfered with their dad's life, and he never asked them for help.

While visiting one Thanksgiving, Mike watched while his dad signed a check that Patricia had filled out. Jim said it was Patricia's payday, and she was now helping him manage his financial affairs. This concerned Mike, so he began to look into things a bit. Mike had noticed that his dad's short-term memory was beginning to slip, and he would frequently forget things he had said or done.

It turned out that Patricia was collecting three and sometimes four $400 paychecks per week, to the tune of $5,000 to $8,000 per month. When Mike confronted his dad about this, he was met with a severe rebuke and was told to mind his own business. Jim had become completely dependent on Patricia to care for him.

He trusted her and was unwilling to part with her, even when confronted with her gross mismanagement and theft. He would admit that she was not perfect, but he would do nothing to jeopardize his relationship with her.

Mike went to his lawyer to find out how to gain some say in his dad's life, for his own good, but he found it to be extremely difficult. His dad would have to sign a release or authorize his son to act as his Power of Attorney, or Jim would have to be deemed incompetent by a court, which was a very expensive and slow process. Jim was a stubborn man and would not have anyone running his life. Because he already perceived his children as trying to interfere with what he knew he wanted, he refused to sign any documents. Mike went to the authorities with all the evidence he had, but they said that as long as he was competent and willingly signing checks, there was nothing they could do.

Mike and Monica wanted to respect their dad's wishes, so, unsure what to do, they stood back and watched while his caregiver drained his accounts. One day Patricia's paycheck bounced. A week later, Mike received a phone call from his dad. Patricia had vanished. Jim was devastated and now had no funds to provide for his care.

This story, although fictional, has played itself out in many lives and will continue to do so as long as people don't understand the laws that govern aging adults. Some families stand back and let Dad run his own life, while others choose to intervene and go down the very painful road of conflict and feel guilty for stripping Dad of his independence. Neither option is pleasant. Here are some safeguards you can put in place to help protect your loved one before it's too late.

KNOW WHAT'S GOING ON IN DAD'S LIFE

You should know who's who in the lives of your loved ones. Meet and talk regularly with their banker, accountant, lawyer, doctors, friends, neighbors, and anyone else who is in regular contact with them. This is especially important if you live far away and don't see them on a regular basis. Be alert for changes that could signal the beginning of a decline. As you evaluate your aging family member's ability to continue living at home without assistance, look at the following signs. Problems in one or more of these areas may call for further assessment and possible part-time help in the home, such as housekeeping, meal services, or medication management.

- Short-term memory loss: forgetting to take medication, forgetting appointments, forgetting meals, balance problems, frequent falls, general unsteadiness
- Difficulty with one or more activities of daily living (ADLs): bathing, eating, toileting, personal hygiene
- Financial mismanagement: unpaid bills, overpaid bills, unawareness of current financial situation
- Getting around: loss of ability to drive safely or secure other means of transportation
- Inability to prepare meals and obtain proper nutrition
- Inability to use a telephone
- Poor judgment: obsession about spending money, not eating wisely, fear of leaving the home, being too trusting or too suspicious of others.

Medical, Financial, and Personal Affairs

As soon as possible, get into a position where you can take control of your loved one's finances should the need arise suddenly. Again, the issue of trust here is huge. Even the closest and most loving families can develop weird feelings when money and control are perceived to be threatened. It is a good idea to have a trusted family friend, accountant, or lawyer involved in conversations and decisions as you work through this. There are many options available.

It is strongly suggested that you discuss these matters in detail with your attorney or CPA. You must understand the laws governing what you can and cannot do, and you must act with integrity so that you don't inadvertently take what isn't yours. Here are some common structures that provide the access you need.

A **Power of attorney** is the authorization to act on someone else's behalf in a legal or business matter. The person authorizing the other to act is the *principal, grantor,* or *donor* and the person authorized to act is the *agent, proxy,* or *attorney-in-fact.* The law requires the agent to be completely honest with and loyal to the principal in their dealings. There are various types of powers of attorney. For example, a healthcare power of attorney empowers the proxy to make medical decisions on the principal's behalf. Other powers may be limited to circumstances in which the grantor is incapacitated. It is best to discuss these issues with an attorney who can guide you in what will best suit your situation.

Advance directives are written statements that define what your wishes are in the event that you are rendered unable to communicate. This may be general or very detailed. It may or may not identify people who can make decisions for you. We recommend obtaining an advance directive as soon as possible. Either you or a trusted friend or family member should have a copy so that if Mom becomes unable to make decisions, her wishes are known and you can legally direct the doctors. Physicians carry a huge liability and are governed by many laws specifying who they can talk to. They have right to refuse to work with even a well-meaning family member who has no legal authority to direct the care of their loved one.

A **living will** is a written document that specifies what medical treatments you desire and what you do not. This too may be very general or quite specific.

One extremely valuable resource to help cover all the bases regarding medical directives and living wills is a booklet called *The Five Wishes*, available without charge at www .arizonahomestead.com. This booklet is for anyone of any age. It will help you determine who you want to make decisions for you, should you lose the ability to do so and specifies advance medical directives stating your wishes for the end of life. It is simple and yet complete, and in Arizona it is respected by all authorities at the same level as any legal document.

Emergency contact numbers: Keep these in convenient places. We even recommend printing them on a small card and carrying them with you (and having your parent do so). Put them in a wallet or your car's glove box in case of an emergency while out alone. Strokes and heart attacks can come out of nowhere and leave a person immediately unable to give the simplest directions.

Funeral arrangements and burial plans: These are much easier to talk about and work through when nobody is dying. Take the time to plan while you are not under the stress of losing or having just lost a loved one. As you approach the subject of caring for your loved ones when they can no longer care for themselves, you must talk, talk, and talk. Talk while you still can.

Long-Term Care Options

There are many options today for long term care. The best approach is to have a strategy ready if and when this decision is upon you. Shop around and know what the options are in your area. When possible, take Mom and Dad with you. Search the Department of Health Services (DHS) website and learn about homes in your zip code. Visit some nursing facilities and make notes of your impressions. You will be much more objective than if you were searching under the pressure of having to place Mom or Dad immediately.

> **As you approach the subject of caring for your loved ones when they can no longer care for themselves, you must talk, talk, and talk. Talk while you still can.**

Discuss what would be important to them if they had to move into long-term care. Cover various scenarios: stroke, hearing loss, vision loss, loss of ability to walk, loss of mental capacity. What would they want in each situation? Nothing is set in stone, but understanding what quality of life looks like from their point of view will take a lot of the mystery out of your decisions when the time comes. In the next chapter we will look at the various options for long-term care and define many of the terms you will encounter.

CHAPTER 2

Long-Term Care Defined

The terms *assisted living, long-term care,* and *skilled nursing* are often used interchangeably, but they are different. As you move into this realm, it's helpful to have good command of a few important terms. These definitions are taken from AZ Statutes: Title 9-Chapter 10-Article 7-701 Definitions which can be found online at www.azdhs.gov/als/hcb/index.htm under the link "Arizona Administrative Code".

TYPES OF LONG-TERM CARE FACILITIES

Independent living applies to facilities where elderly individuals live who can mostly care for themselves, but because of the frailty that comes with aging they wish to be in a more secure environment. Usually a few meals are prepared and the person has his own kitchenette. He is responsible for housekeeping, laundry, and personal medications, and he completes all activities of daily living on his own.

An **assisted-living facility** is a step up from independent living. Assisted living differs depending on the state in which you live. In Arizona it is defined as a *residential care institution, including adult foster care, that provides or contracts to provide supervisory care services, personal care services or directed care services on a continuing basis.* These facilities are either homes (ten or fewer residents) or centers (eleven or more residents). They cannot perform ongoing nursing activities such as maintaining IVs. In many instances, services can be provided by a home health agency in an assisted-living facility if the patient doesn't require 24-hour supervision. These facilities can generally care for residents requiring some level of assistance all the way through hospice.

A **skilled nursing facility,** also known as a nursing care institution or nursing home, is a health care institution providing inpatient beds or resident beds and nursing services to persons who need nursing services on a continuing basis but who do not require hospital care or direct daily care from a physician. These facilities can care for all levels of physical and cognitive decline.

LEVELS OF CARE

Within assisted living, there are various levels of care for which specific rules and regulations apply. Applicable statutes are quoted in italics.

Supervisory care services means general supervision, including daily awareness of resident functioning and continuing needs, the ability to intervene in a crisis and assistance in the self-administration of prescribed medications. This level is limited to supervision without hands-on assistance. Administering medications is not permitted at this level, and neither is caring for a confused person unable to self-direct.

Personal care services means assistance with activities of daily living that can be performed by persons without professional skills or professional training and includes the coordination or provision of intermittent nursing services and the administration of medications and treatments by a nurse who is licensed pursuant to Title 32, Chapter 15, or as otherwise provided by law. This is basically all levels of nonmedical physical assistance.

Directed care services means programs and services, including supervisory and personal care services, provided to persons who are incapable of recognizing danger, summoning assistance, expressing need or making basic care decisions. This category accounts for dementia and cognitive disabilities. It is the most comprehensive care.

WHO'S CARING FOR YOUR LOVED ONE?

A number of different levels of trained staff will be caring for your loved one. Most people requiring 24/7 care do not need an entire skilled nursing staff, which comes with a very high price tag. Instead, in assisted living situations, what a person needs most is the presence of people who can help with daily living activities and who can recognize issues that may need attention. These are some of the professionals who serve in assisted-living facilities.

> **In assisted living, what a person needs most is someone who can help with daily activities and who can recognize issues that need attention.**

Certified caregiver: Arizona has a certification for a caregiver offering services in an assisted-living situation. Caregivers are certified at three levels, corresponding with the care levels defined above: supervisory, personal, and directed. These people are trained in the specific tasks entrusted to them. These are mainly assisting with daily living, preparing meals, doing laundry, and recognizing danger signs, in addition to special training in dispensing medication. A certified caregiver must be at least eighteen years old. Anyone left alone with patients must be at least twenty-one years old and certified at all the home's levels of care. All staff must supply proof of freedom from tuberculosis on an annual basis, and keep their CPR and first aid training updated. They must have a fingerprint clearance card on record.

Assistant caregiver: This person must be at least sixteen years old. She must be under the direct supervision of a manager or caregiver at all times and may assist in all aspects of care except for bathing, toileting, transfers, self-administration of medications, medication administration, and nursing services.

Certified Nurse Assistant (CNA): This is a position overseen by the nursing department. A CNA holds a license that must be kept current. CNAs are not allowed to dispense medications without a special caregiver bridge.

Licensed Manager: Managers of assisted-living facilities are licensed by the Arizona Board of Examiners of Nursing Care Institution Administrators and Assisted Living Facility Managers (NCIA). They should have a good understanding of the laws that govern the industry, a working knowledge of the nursing skills they manage on a daily basis, and skills in working with people. Managers are generally on call 24/7 and deserve a great deal of respect for the enormous responsibility they bear.

Licensed Practical Nurse (LPN): This is a nurse trained in routine nursing care who is allowed to perform complex tasks under the direction of a physician or registered nurse.

Registered Nurse (RN): An RN must pass an exam and be licensed by the state board of nursing.

Nurse Practitioner: This is an RN who has been trained to a higher level and is able to take on many activities normally carried out by a physician, such as diagnosing and prescribing treatments. This is a very valuable role in assisted living situations, as these practitioners are much more hands-on and up-to-date on the issues facing the aging population. Often their entire clientele is elderly, and they come around to see them in their places of residence.

STATE AND PRIVATE AGENCIES

The **Arizona Long-term Care System (ALTCS)** is an Arizona Medicaid program under the Arizona Health Care Cost Containment System (AHCCCS). ALTCS pays for long- term care costs for those individuals and families who qualify, not only in nursing homes, but also in assisted-living homes and centers with whom they are contracted. ALTCS also covers costs of services in the senior's own home. To apply for ALTCS or to find more information, go to www.azahcccs.gov.

The **Pima Council on Aging (PCOA)** is a nonprofit advocacy organization that offers support to seniors needing health care. Learn more about how they can serve you at www.pcoa.org.

Adult Protective Services (APS) is a division of the Arizona Department of Economic Security. This is the agency to contact should you encounter abuse, neglect, or exploitation of a vulnerable or elderly adult. Many times an elderly adult will be living alone and unable to adequately care for himself, in which case APS can come in and help him negotiate a more appropriate living situation. They can also provide legal support and advice concerning powers of attorney, wills, trusts, and other fiduciary services. You can learn more about APS at www.azdes.gov /aaa/programs/aps. To report any suspicion of abuse or neglect, call 1-877-SOS-ADULT (1-877-767-2385).

The **Department of Health Services (DHS)** Division of Licensing Services/Assisted Living is the government department that licenses all assisted living facilities. DHS sends out surveyors who do annual inspections and follow up on complaints submitted by individuals or anonymously. Their website is www.azdhs.gov/als.

The **ombudsman program** is a division of the Arizona State Legislature. The ombudsman serves as an advocate for the elderly. If there is a situation that you cannot resolve with a loved one, a care center, or any aspect of your care journey, you can contact the long- term care ombudsman's office, and they will help you to find solutions. They can be contacted through www.azdes.gov and www.azdhs.gov.

There are two types of **referral and placement agencies**. One group consists of large national companies that subcontract with agents in the area. These companies usually have a large Internet presence and do most of their business on the Web. The other group is made up of smaller individually-owned agencies that network with hospitals and rehab centers in addition to marketing their services in other ways.

Both types of agents collect information from clients seeking care and generally do not charge the client a fee. They contract with homes and centers who agree to pay a fee for any resident placed in the facility. Locally-owned and operated agencies tend to be more familiar with the homes and centers. Beware of agencies that cast the care industry in a bad light and promote fear and mistrust. Many of these will refer you to the home that pays the highest fee, regardless of quality of care.

Hospice is a Medicare-funded program that assists patients who have a life expectancy of six months or less. Various organizations provide hospice services, and it is up to the patient and the family to choose. Providers may vary widely in the types of services they offer, so be sure to interview several hospice organizations before making a decision.

CHAPTER 3

Finding a Home: The Process

Finding an assisted-living situation for your family member should be done carefully to reduce stress on everyone involved. A step-by-step process will help you to be objective and thorough in making your decision. It is important to involve Mom in the process whenever possible. When this isn't possible, be sure to get input from everyone involved who knows her well and understands her preferences. Here is an outline of the process you might follow, but you will want to add and change steps as your situation warrants.

Quality of life: What is most important to you and Dad? Decide what is most important to his quality of life. Do this before you begin looking, so that you won't lose sight of these considerations during the process. You may be dazzled by a number of extras that really don't contribute to Dad's most important needs.

Conducting a search: Look on the DHS website and find homes in your zip code or area of preference (www.azdhs .gov/als). Call and visit as many facilities as you can in order to get a feel for what is available. If you wish to use the services of a referral agent, do so. As you conduct your search, you can go to the following website and find how each home and center has fared during their annual state survey: www.azdhs.gov/als/hcb/index.htm. Click on "Facility Search Including Inspection Reports." You will need the name or address of the specific facility you are interested in.

Understanding the Survey: All state-licensed facilities must pass an initial survey or inspection before obtaining a license. After that, they are inspected either annually or every two years. The home is issued a new license once the application is submitted and fees are paid, and then the state surveyor is free to come and inspect any time during the next year. If the home is found to be deficiency-free, the inspection is waived for the following year.

As with all systems, this is designed to bring accountability to the service providers and verify that they are operating within the intent of the law. Surveys are like tax audits. Many of us would not do well on a tax audit if we had no warning. We may not keep our accounts completely up to date throughout the year, but if we are responsible, we manage to catch up by April 15. If we are honest all year and keep reasonable notes, tax time is not such a challenge. Surveys are much like this. Keep in mind that surveyors are human and vary in their personalities. Some are more forgiving than others. Some give suggestions where others might issue a deficiency. They operate within a set of legal boundaries, but a fairly wide area is open to subjective interpretation.

Kinds of deficiencies: The DHS website will tell you which homes have deficiencies and which do not, as well as which homes have had penalties or civil violations. It is very difficult to complete a survey with no deficiencies, so you are right to be impressed when a home manages that. That being said, however, you need to know that, just as it's possible to cheat on your taxes, there are ways to be deficiency-free at inspection time and substandard the rest of the year. Just because the home has no deficiencies doesn't mean things are in order all the time. Don't let survey results be your only guide to the quality of the home.

When you're touring, look for signs that all is in order. Appendix 1 has a list of things you can check that will indicate whether the home functions at that standard all year round. Understand that some homes are administratively excellent but don't provide the warm and caring environment that will maximize the residents' quality of life. Look for the right balance of formal and informal qualities.

If you visit a home and feel good about it but find that it has deficiencies, consider what they are and how they were reconciled. Discuss the issues with administrators and staff. If they give you satisfactory answers, you can feel reassured. Often a mark or a citation results in a much stronger home. Deficiencies can be seen as educational tools for the home. With improvements in the quality of administrators and staff, problems can be resolved and the home environment improved.

OVERALL MANAGEMENT

The management of a facility is affected as much by behind-the-scenes levels of management as by day-to-day operations. These should be considered in your selection.

Owner Involvement

It is important to understand the role of the home's owner. There is a difference between the mom-and-pop operation where the owner is there 24/7 and does a lot of the work and the large corporation where the owner lives elsewhere and oversees from a distance. Either scenario can work, but you must adjust your expectations accordingly. Generally, homes where owners are involved are stronger overall. The buck stops with the owner. If she is available, approachable, and visible, this is a huge plus. No one loves your kids like you do, no one cares for your money like you do, and no one will care for a business like the owner. He may not pull shifts or provide actual care, but you should consider it a red flag if he is not engaged in any way.

Financial Viability

Don't hesitate to ask questions related to the business aspect of the facility. They may be the greatest provider in town, but if they go bankrupt the week you move Mom in, it's a bad situation. While you may not be able to look at account statements, feel free to ask questions such as Have you ever missed a payroll? Do you have liability insurance? What is your staffing ratio? Does the home adhere to the current code requirements? Later in this chapter, we will discuss costs involved in running a home and define reasonable expectations.

THE REFERRAL AGENT

A referral agent can be a tremendous help, especially when you need to find a place quickly. Agents are in and out of facilities all the time. They tend to know what various places offer and what types of residents live there. They're in business to find a good fit for your loved one. Your understanding of the agent's role will empower you and enable you to make the best use of her time and talent.

At present, the referral agent system in Arizona is largely unregulated. Here are the limited regulations that exist.

- Homes must have a contract with anyone to whom they pay a referral fee, and each agent or agency develops its own contract.
- The state prohibits any additional fee from being passed on to the resident if a family chooses to use a referral agent.

The agent does not charge the family but instead charges the facility for each placement. Some referral agents tour with the family and provide genuine guidance and support. Others merely hand out a list of phone numbers and the family tours alone. A few might assist with discharge from the hospital, transportation to the facility, and other aspects of the transition.

Hospitals and rehabilitation centers generally will not directly refer a patient to an individual facility in order to avoid potential future liability. Referral agents are therefore the first to receive a name of someone looking for placement. Homes not listed with the referral agent you choose will not be shown.

UNDERSTANDING THE COSTS INVOLVED

Costs are a critical subject to discuss. You might spent between $2,000 and $7,000 a month for one bedroom (sometimes a shared bedroom) in a house or other facility, so the fees can seem rather steep. It is important to understand what that fee has to pay for.

Lois and Frank's Story

The strain was beginning to show on the faces of the five adult children caring for their aging parents. Frank and Lois had been married for almost 15 years. He was 97 and had lost his wife of 52 years 20 years earlier. He had two sons. Lois was 88. She had been married for 20 years before her husband was killed in a car accident. She had not remarried until she met Frank 16 years earlier. Lois had a son and two daughters.

They had been very good for each other. He suffered from a very slowly progressing Parkinson's disease that was well controlled with medication. Lois was in very good health except for a slight cholesterol problem that she managed with a good diet and a few pills. It was clear the couple loved each other dearly.

Frank's greatest desire was to be allowed to age and die in the home 60 years. He had watched his first wife suffer in a nursing home as cancer slowly robbed her of life before finally releasing her from this world. He had watched helplessly and felt completely powerless to change anything as he was tossed to and fro in the wild sea of the medical system.

Life was ideal until the accident. As Frank's Parkinson's gradually became worse, Lois had taken on more and more of the role of a caregiver. Finally one day about three months ago, Frank fell. Fortunately nothing was broken, but he was in a great deal of pain and unable to get out of bed. Lois's blood pressure had been borderline and over the past year had crept up to dangerous levels. She maintained a healthy diet and was very good about taking her pills, but the stress of caring for him and seeing the pain he was suffering became too much, and a week after Frank came home, Lois suffered a stroke. After two weeks in the hospital and another two weeks in rehab, she was ready to come home.

The family had taken turns caring for Frank while they researched their options. It had been six weeks since his fall. Both parents were enrolled in hospice, so they had the support of hospice nurses and shower aides coming to their home. But that didn't begin to touch the 24/7 need for assistance with toileting, meals, housekeeping, and other care. It was a considerable challenge to navigate around the tiny old house using wheelchairs and walkers.

Tensions were high and tempers were short. The cost of round-the-clock care was nearly $15,000 a month, and though all five kids wanted to do what was absolutely best for their parents, they couldn't afford to keep that up for more than a couple of months without throwing everyone into bankruptcy.

Frank and Lois's children were learning a very expensive lesson about the costs of in-home health care. To put it in perspective, paying for 24-hour care in your own home will cost a minimum of $7,300 a month. That's $10 an hour times 24 hours a day times 365 days, divided by 12 months, and it's hard to find someone for $10 an hour. In addition to that, you're paying the mortgage or rent, utilities, taxes, groceries, and so on. Then you still have to manage the caregivers. When they call in sick, you're on the hook.

Another option is to hire an agency to provide care, but then the price will be $13 to $30 an hour, or $14,000 or more a month above basic living expenses. So $3,000 to $5,000 a month for housing, food, and care looks more reasonable. Furthermore, there are many homes where Granddad will receive much better care than you may find from an agency, and the homes are almost always wheelchair-accessible.

Three thousand dollars for a private room is a very reasonable price. The costs are considerable on the provider's side. Staffing accounts for at least 50 percent of what a home brings in. The facility must pay for mortgage and utilities, liability insurance, taxes, the endless maintenance and upgrades necessary to maintain a healthy environment, and empty rooms and a referral fee to get them filled, not to mention groceries and other supplies for the residents. Three thousand dollars each for ten residents is just about the minimum required to provide the quality care that most of us want for our loved ones.

As you shop for a home, cheaper rooms can be very appealing, and these facilities might provide outstanding care, but you must find out where corners are being cut. Is the staff paid adequately? Is there a high staff turnover? What is the ratio of staff to residents? What is the menu like? Is the facility maintained adequately? Is the owner working around the clock and ready to burn out? Often a home can provide excellent care on a shoestring because the owner or manager is very thrifty and conscientious. Conversely, a home can be overpriced and still cut the same corners.

> **When cost is an issue, you can provide services that the home cannot afford to offer, such as bringing in extra goodies, taking Mom out, or sending in a sitter to play games or otherwise provide extra attention.**

Be observant, investigate, and know what you're paying for. Know where you can fill in on your loved one's behalf to enhance his or her wellbeing. This might be supplementing the menu with homemade goodies you know Mom loves, or bringing Dad a stash of cans of Dr Pepper. You might send a sitter in to play favorite games or read to him. You can take Mom to the beauty salon once a week if she would enjoy that. There are many ways to improve Grandma's situation over what the facility provides. The key is clarifying your expectations, as will be discussed in the next chapter.

Important Consideration for This Season of Life

This book would not be complete without a segment on the significance of the final few years of life. As an individual approaches the end, every day becomes a huge percentage of the rest of her life. When considering what is best for your loved one, please see that these final days, months, years are as comfortable as humanly possible. This is not the time to save money. If someone you love is in an unsatisfactory situation, don't let him stay there just to use up the cost of the 30 days' notice or for other financial reasons. No amount of money is worth your loved one's having to suffer during the final days of life. If you feel the end is near, a few hundred dollars a month difference between a very high quality place and a budget place that is inadequately staffed will not amount to much in exchange for a pleasant journey to the finish line.

WHEN THE MONEY RUNS OUT

For many people facing long-term care, money will be a problem. Perhaps it just simply isn't there. When the money is gone, ALTCS, funded by Medicaid, is a viable option. In fact, it is only an option when the money is entirely gone. Any income, Social Security, or pension payments are turned over to the state, as are all assets. The state then takes over payment for all long-term care services.

Private pay will almost always secure a better environment. When government money is involved, bureaucracy increases. This is the case with ALTCS. As soon as Uncle Sam pays the bill, you can expect greater scrutiny of what goes on. This doesn't necessarily mean that the quality will be better. It means that more time will be devoted to "proving" that standards are being met, which is not the same thing as providing quality care.

ALTCS pays a flat rates for residents qualifying at three different levels of care. The monthly rate varies, but it is somewhere around $2,000 a month. Homes providing more than two ALTCS beds are hard-pressed to staff adequately and provide the standard of care most of us would want. However, when money is absent, this is certainly an option.

Understand that an ALTCS placement will generally mean a shared bedroom and one caregiver for ten residents, regardless of level of care. When this is the case, know the numbers and adjust your expectations accordingly. The family can make up for a lot in these situations. If the home can meet the resident's basic needs of food, housing, supervision, cleanliness, and medication management, the family can come in and meet the need for social interaction, activity, and entertainment. The family can also pay for a companion to come in and sit with the resident, take them out if they are able, play games, read books or just provide company.

With ALTCS you limit your options dramatically, because many homes choose not to accept ALTCS funds in order to avoid the added complexity and inconvenience, lower revenues, and increased scrutiny that come with them.

Long-Term Care Insurance

Long-term care insurance is great if you have it. Most ten-bedroom homes qualify for this type of insurance. Generally the home completes some paperwork, you pay the bill, and the insurance company reimburses you. This can take a huge weight off the family by greatly reducing, if not eliminating, the overwhelming costs associated with long-term care. Keep in mind that most insurance companies pay after the service is rendered, while most facilities charge in advance. Therefore you will want to be prepared to pay up front and receive the reimbursement later. A number of companies offer this insurance. There is a list on our website at www.arizonahomestead.com.

Caring for Mom at Home

People often opt to try to take care of a family member at home. This can be a great option. We have seen some of our own residents go through rehabilitation from an accident or injury and return home to live very happily with a family who can meet their needs. Maybe there are grandkids or stay-at-home spouses available so that Grandpa isn't home alone but has the company and supervision he needs to be happy and content.

Be aware, however, that coming home can also lead to disaster. When families try to care for their aging loved ones at home, they are often neglected more than would be tolerated in even the worst of care facilities. It's not that the families don't care, but the reality is that we live in a busy society where both husband and wife frequently work outside the home or are involved in activities requiring them to be out of the house.

Maybe you know someone who says, "Oh, I take care of my mom at home. She can't walk, but I just tell her to stay in her chair until I get home [maybe eight hours later] and she does fine." This is *not* fine. A care-home owner would go to jail if they took this attitude. Be reasonable if you want to care for your parent at home. Know what you can and cannot do. Know what they need and be sure you can provide it.

Another consideration when caring for family at home is the health of the caregiver. A spouse can completely ruin her own health while caring for the other. A study conducted through Ohio State University and the University of North Carolina produced strong evidence that the continuing stress of providing in-home care can cause severe, long-term damage to the immune system of the caregiver. For more information, and some very interesting reading, go to www.researchnews.osu.edu/search.htm and enter caregiver fatigue in the search box.

> **When procuring in-home care services, find agencies that have safeguards in place, such as training, fingerprint screening, and background checks for their caregivers.**

Many agencies send a caregiver into your home to help out. If what you need is supervision or assistance for a few hours a day, this can be an excellent solution. The cost will be comparable to 24-hour care in a facility, and you can still have Mom close by. Many long-term care insurance policies will cover this type of service.

Be aware that in Arizona, agencies that provide home caregivers are unregulated. You need to be diligent and observant. Find agencies that have safeguards in place, such as training, fingerprint screening, and background checks for their caregivers.

In the next chapter we will discuss how to function in the assisted-living system.

CHAPTER 4

Functioning in the System

ENTERING THE SYSTEM

The process of moving a loved one into an assisted-living facility varies widely from family to family and from situation to situation. Only the family, responsible party, or intimate friend can decide the best way to help an individual make that transition. Moving into a long-term care setting can be a breath of fresh air if one is coming from an institutional setting or anywhere that basic needs are not being met. It can also entail an enormous sense of loss if moving from a home where one has lived for many years. Fortunately, there are many good options out there. The transition does not have to mean life is over.

> **Moving into long-term care can entail an enormous sense of loss of freedom, privacy, independence, space, and property. It is important for all involved to be sympathetic toward the feelings and fears of the person moving.**

Regardless of your individual situation, it's very important for all involved to be sympathetic toward the feelings and fears of the person moving into long-term care. Feelings of loss of freedom, privacy, independence, space, and property can be huge. These are very real fears when a vulnerable adult places herself in the care of complete strangers, many of whom look different from the people she is used to.

Whatever can be done to alleviate those fears should be done. We always suggest that the manager or owner of the facility meet the prospective resident so that the family has a face to associate with the new home. This can set Mom at ease and alleviate many fears. Also, if possible, bring the resident into the home for lunch or an activity in order to see who their new housemates and caregivers will be. Not only will this set people at ease if they like what they see, it can also prevent a poor placement or poor fit into a community that is not going to work. As a home owner, I welcome this almost as much as the good fit because of the problems that occur when a resident moves in who is not appropriate for our setting.

Every home and community has its own personality. Even in the three homes that we own, we see this among staff and residents. One place is a sanctuary for one person while for another it can be completely intolerable. Encourage the prospective resident to be as involved as possible in the transition.

KNOW YOUR FAMILY MEMBER

We find there are basically three types of residents. You will know which category fits your loved one, and thinking about that ahead of time will help you in your relationship with the facility and will contribute to your loved one's happiness. Every human being deserves to be treated with dignity and respect. There is never a valid excuse, regardless of how difficult an individual may be, for neglect, abuse, or mistreatment in any care setting. Here are the three general types of assisted-living residents.

Never happy no matter what: You try and try to make the person happy, but they will have none of it!. The bed is always too hard or too saggy, the chair is all wrong, and the food is just *How do you expect me to eat this slop?* The house is either too hot or too cold. The caregiver has no common sense and neither does the person's own son or daughter. Nobody can ever get anything right. Complaining almost seems to be the only thing that makes him happy. This category includes both the confused and the truly paranoid as well as the alert and oriented who are just plain cranky or difficult.

What you must know about this person in the long-term care system is that they are very likely targets for abuse or neglect. If this is your loved one, it is very important that you communicate frequently with the facility staff and make sure that you all understand the nature of the resident. If the person is a habitual complainer, let the staff know you understand that, but at the same time be alert to signs of abuse or neglect. Caregivers are human and may easily overlook the person who is likely to ruin their day. That person, however, is a vulnerable adult and deserves to be cared for and looked after. Find a few things that you know your loved one truly appreciates and make every effort to supply those things.

Completely content no matter what: This is the person who is very easy to love. No one can do wrong. They are completely understanding and tolerant of uncomfortable beds, poor chairs, and lousy food. They understand nobody's perfect and extend grace to the clumsy caregiver, forgetful son or daughter, or obnoxious fellow resident. (This one is probably married to the person in the preceding paragraph, by the way.) They smile and say thank you and are rarely a trouble. This is the person every care home wants to take care of. This person also can be overlooked and neglected simply because she is not a squeaky wheel. If this is your loved one, encourage her to communicate her wants and needs. You also should feel free to tell the staff about needs that Mom feels comfortable sharing with you but not with them.

Happy as long as a few key needs are met: This is the category most of us fit into. For the most part, if a few key expectations are met, we can live contentedly and get along. For most of us, though, without certain things, life can really stink. Maybe it's that fresh-ground cup of coffee right when you wake up, or the afternoon martini you've been enjoying for the past sixty years. We have developed a brief quality-of-life questionnaire (Appendix 2) that helps to identify these core needs. If the home you're considering doesn't have something like this in place, you might want to complete the form so that your expectations are clear and in writing. In the beginning, follow up frequently to make sure the routines in place are taking these things into account.

COMMUNICATION AND DEVELOPING A TEAM

Caring for Mom Once Settled

A mistake many make is thinking that once you have secured a location for your loved one you can now become disengaged. Not so! It is very important to accompany your loved one through the system. Just as no one will love your children the way you do and no one will care about your money the way you do, no one will love your Mom and Dad the way you do. That doesn't mean that they cannot take care of them as well as you would, it just means that even in the best of facilities, people are fallible, and important things can get overlooked. The more people there are who focus on Mom, the better off she will be. Any good facility will welcome your insights, suggestions and overall input. Also, your presence will most likely result in improved staff performance overall.

Building a Relationship with the Caregiving Team

The best way to ensure quality care is to build a relationship with the caregiving team. Every business and social network has both its angels and its demons. Please, for your family member's sake, be an angel in the system in which you find yourself. This will make a huge difference in the way people respond to you and Mom.

> **Be an angel in the system in which you find yourself. This will make a huge difference in the way people will respond to you and your family member.**

A good relationship with the facility depends primarily on three things: honest communication, kind communication, and respectful communication. Careful communication will do more than any team of lawyers and doctors to promote the comfort and care of your family member. Respect the team as a group of people who are generally underpaid for the value they offer. They do what they do mostly because they genuinely care about the people they care for and reap great nonmonetary rewards for their work. But there are exceptions to every rule. If you see problems arising, waste no time in addressing them calmly and chances are they will never reach crisis level.

THE COMMUNICATION TRIANGLE

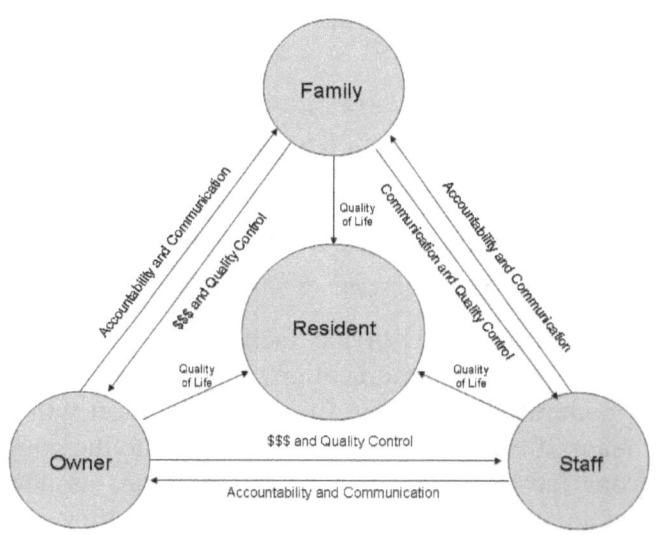

We designed this triangle as a way to see how the communication needs to flow and where the accountability lines are in the effort to provide the highest quality of life possible to our residents. We are all in this business for that one reason. This balance must always be kept in place. Sometimes the staff may play the family against the owner, or the family may pit the resident against the staff, or there might be some other dysfunctional scenario. The only way the resident's quality of life will be maintained is if the lines of communication are functioning well.

You may want to use the triangle as a tool to initiate communication with the manager or owner of the facility. Find out what she does to keep the lines open and what accountability structures are in place. If you have a problem with a caregiver or another resident, address it with the manager. If that doesn't bring about the results you need, what does the facility want you to do next?

In our homes, we make ourselves available to ensure that such problems are corrected. It works very well. The manager doesn't always have the resources or the authority to make the corrections, so the team should include an active owner or an administrator who carries the authority to solve problems.

HOW THINGS WORK

Certain rules and regulations govern assisted-living facilities. Here are a few things you should know about what the law requires.

Tuberculosis and Flu

Before you move Dad into an assisted-living facility, you will need to provide proof that he is free from tuberculosis. This can be determined by a chest x-ray or a skin test. The form signed by the doctor or nurse must state that he is free from TB. It cannot merely say *no active disease* or something of that nature. Be sure to notify your doctor or hospital staff that you need this before moving your relative. The test must be repeated on an annual basis to ensure ongoing freedom from TB.

The facility is required by law to make flu and pneumococcal vaccines available to its residents annually. If you and Mom decide to forgo these vaccines, you will need to notify the facility in writing.

The Service Plan

Within fourteen days of move-in, according to Arizona law, assisted-living facilities must prepare a service plan, also called a care plan, outlining the nature of the care the facility will provide.

This is done by the manager, by a registered nurse, or by a nurse practitioner. In the case of a directed-care resident, it must be done by at least an RN. There is generally an additional charge to you for this service, and you will be asked to participate and sign the care plan.

The plan defines exactly what services the home will provide to assist with medication and activities of daily living. The law states that the plan must be updated whenever there are significant changes, or upon return if resident goes to the hospital. There is usually a charge each time the plan is updated.

The Chain of Command

In an assisted-living situation, the staff must abide by *doctor's orders*. These are maintained on a form stating what medications and treatments the resident can and must receive, dosages, times, and any special instructions. Some meds are ordered regularly, such as blood pressure medicine; others are PRN (as needed), such as Tylenol for a headache. The facility is obligated to follow doctor's orders.

Often a family member will want to make changes or hold a medication. They may just disagree with the physician. Even if you hold medical power of attorney, you may not instruct the caregiver or staff to violate doctor's orders. If you wish to make a change, discuss it with the doctor, who can then issue new orders. The staff cannot give any medication that is not listed on the orders, and they must give those that are ordered. Because of potential drug interactions, the use of alcohol must be approved by doctor's order as well.

ADVANCE DIRECTIVES

DNR: The Do-Not-Resuscitate Order

When you place Dad in long-term care, you will be asked about his end-of-life wishes and whether he wants to receive heroic measures should his heart stop or should he require life support.

One option is *Full Code*, meaning that if his heart stops, he wants all measures taken to revive him. Another is *Do Not Resuscitate (DNR)*, meaning that if his heart stops, he does not want to be resuscitated but wants to be allowed to allow nature to take its course.

An orange DNR form will be kept on file for those who do not wish to have extreme measures taken to keep them alive. Naturally, this doesn't mean that if a person is choking on a hot dog, the staff will stand by and let her die or that they won't call the paramedics if it looks like she's having a stroke. It merely means that if the staff or paramedics see that a person's heart has stopped, they will not perform CPR or otherwise try to bring her back.

The Living Will and Related Issues

It is extremely important to find out Dad's end-of-life wishes while he can still tell you what they are. Many resources are available to help you do this. Medical and financial powers of attorney should be obtained in the event that Dad loses his mental faculties. Your family member may assign someone power of attorney, but the power to make decisions for him only exists should he not be able to make decisions for himself.

A valuable resource that is respected by all authorities in Arizona is *The Five Wishes*. This walks you through each major area of decision-making. Every adult should have a copy and should keep it updated in case of emergency. Be sure to have it signed and notarized so there is no question as to its validity. *The*

Five Wishes can be purchased at www.agingwithdignity.org or you can obtain a free one through our website at www .arizonahomestead.com.

EXPECTATIONS AND QUALITY OF LIFE

What Is Reasonable?

It is important to identify some core things that are necessary to your loved one's happiness before you select a home. Otherwise you might be swayed into a situation that ultimately will not suit you. It is important to communicate these things at the outset.

No facility can be everything to everyone, but any home can cater to a few important things for each resident if they make it a priority. For example, maybe hot coffee at 5:00 AM every morning is critical to Dad's having a good day, but Bingo on Thursday is not at all to his taste. Perhaps Uncle Joe craves peanut butter and jelly with an ice-cold Coke at 2:00 PM, but he really doesn't like Sunday worship Another resident might say that Sunday worship is the only thing that keeps him going from week to week, but he hates coffee and only gets hungry at mealtimes. Identify some things that are important to your loved one and tell the staff about them. It is not unreasonable to expect the home to accommodate you.

What to Expect from a Large Center

Larger centers may not be able to give Mom as much personal attention, but it can happen, and they can offer many things smaller homes cannot. You will have a bigger job of communicating with caregivers on a larger staff. You may need to take on the role of quality-of-life manager and see to it that friends and family visit and help Dad feel secure and cared for.

Larger centers can offer a greater array of activities, such as transportation to shopping centers and other places, regular recreation, and restaurant-style dining.

Certain services are perfectly reasonable and should be offered by any assisted-living facility. You can expect the home to do the following.

- Accurately manage medications and treatments
- Maintain a clean, odor-free environment
- Serve balanced, nutritious, tasty meals
- Respect the residents' dignity and rights and treat them with kindness and common sense
- Attempt to incorporate residents' personal interests and tastes into the home's activities and menus
- Comply with all applicable rules and regulations
- Be receptive to communication and willing to solve problems.

It is not reasonable to expect the facility to be perfect or to lavish attention on your loved one. He may not get one-on-one attention if you aren't paying a one-on-one price. Caregivers cannot be expected to perform personal tasks for a resident beyond assistance with defined activities of daily living. Residents may not be able to request individualized meals.

Such services can be requested ahead of time, and the provider, the resident, and the family can agree on what is expected. Personal attention is available at the right price. If you are willing to spend $8,000 to $10,000 a month, you can see to it that your loved one receives individual attention, personal services, and a varied menu of choices at meals.

ABUSE

When to Be Truly Concerned: Signs of Neglect and Abuse

Neglect and abuse can and do occur in assisted-living facilities, and it's important to be able to recognize some signs, especially if your loved one is confused, difficult to manage, or unable to communicate. Some of the most likely targets of abuse are demanding, unkind, and uncooperative residents.

It's often hard to pin down incidents of actual abuse. One of the first signs of dementia is paranoia. Residents who are confused often become fearful and imagine things that are not true. It is up to you to distinguish the real from the merely perceived. Here are some signs to look for.

- Outright accusations. These need to be taken in context.
- Bruising or burns that look suspicious.
- Bedsores in otherwise healthy residents, except toward the end of life as the body loses the ability to heal itself.
- Psychological changes such as fear of abandonment or unusual attachment to a certain person.

Legal Responsibilities Regarding Abuse

Every care environment is governed by laws that obligate caregivers and staff to report any abuse they witness or suspect, even by visitors and family members. If an employee witnesses or suspects abuse, he has a legal obligation to report it to Adult Protective Services. Failure to do so can result in fines and even arrest. APS then conducts an investigation and helps to resolve problems that might have triggered the alleged abuse.

Often families have disagreements, and tempers can flair. You need to know that it is always unacceptable to use abusive speech or actions toward a vulnerable adult. Withholding medication and treatments is considered negligent, and the family cannot fail to supply the facility with the means to carry out doctor's orders.

When to Call in Hospice

Hospice does not mean you are going to die today or next week, or even this year. The general guideline for enrolling in hospice care is that there is a reasonable chance you could pass away within the next six months. Generally speaking, enrolling in hospice says *I'm done fighting and trying to get better. I'm ready to let nature take its course. Please keep me comfortable.*

The hospice organization will do an evaluation at the request of the primary-care doctor and determine if the person is eligible. Weight loss, failure to thrive, terminal diagnoses, chronic heart failure, stroke, or high risk of another heart attack are some of the things that might make one eligible.

There are very good reasons for enrolling your loved one. Hospice generally pays for all pain and palliative or comfort medications as well as incontinence supplies and added care assistance, such as a shower aide. Hospice provides for an RN to visit the resident as often as necessary for his comfort and well-being. This added medical attention often leads to significant recovery, and many people are taken off hospice because they begin to improve and even thrive.

Some hospice agencies send out activity or companion aides who will play games or just sit with your loved one to meet the need for social interaction. Most hospice agencies assign a social worker to act as an advocate with the medical system and the management of the facility. Hospice can provide chaplains of all faiths for spiritual support.

These people not only care for the dying person but also offer grief counseling and coping support for the family and caregivers. Most of us want to be able to die with dignity and with minimal pain. On hospice, medications are made available to alleviate pain and anxiety, allowing the patient to pass peacefully. Without hospice, it can be difficult to obtain palliative medications in sufficient dosages to make the patient comfortable.

What Hospice Is Not

Hospice is not a death sentence. For instance, if you are in hospice for terminal cancer and you get pneumonia, you may certainly opt to be treated for it. If you are on hospice for failure to thrive and you fall and break a hip, you can choose to be taken immediately to the hospital and be treated or you can remain where you are and receive comfort care. Once you decide to go to the hospital, you might be discharged from hospice, but you can be readmitted later. You will never be refused treatment because you are on hospice care, but certain treatments, such as physical therapy, can disqualify you from the program.

CHAPTER 5

Ending Your Long-Term Care Experience

You might end your long-term care experience for any of several reasons, such as the following.

- Your loved one may improve and be able to return to living independently.
- You may be unhappy with the current facility or otherwise decide that a different facility will better meet your loved one's needs.
- Your loved one passes away and services are no longer needed.

There are some helpful things to know that will make the transition less stressful.

RETURNING HOME

What a joy when this happens! We have had people in our care go from hospice to thriving to moving back home.

There are certain things to think about if this occurs. Know what your contract says regarding termination of the agreement. Most places require a thirty-day written notice. It will make everyone's life easier if you do this, even if the contract does not require it. If you move out with less than thirty days' notice, the home may continue to charge for those days, because they don't have enough time to advertise the room and get it filled. This is not unreasonable. Once you have given your notice and moved out, you should be reimbursed any unused fees and your security deposit, if any, within thirty days.

MOVING FROM ONE FACILITY TO ANOTHER

Moving between facilities can be a touchy thing. Moving from rehab into an assisted-living facility or from a lower level of care into a higher level is commonplace and need not involve conflict. Moving because you are unhappy brings an added need for tact and etiquette. In either case, to ensure the smoothest transition possible, communicate very clearly to both the home you are leaving and the one you are moving the resident into. Sometimes people want to avoid conflict, so they leave without notice. This is not a good strategy. It is always better to stick with clear communication. If you are concerned about the reaction of the staff upon your communication or feel they may talk you into staying, bring along an advocate who can stand up to them and who is not as emotionally involved. It can be a very sensitive issue, but you will better serve the needs of your loved one by doing things properly and being up front in your communications.

- Submit a letter of termination that includes your name, the date, the date of the move, and if you want to include it, the reason for the move. If you choose not to give thirty days' notice, be prepared to pay for the remaining days or there may be difficulties down the line.

- Obtain copies of the care plan, signed doctor's orders, documentation of freedom from TB, all medications, lab reports as needed, and the original orange DNR (which should accompany the resident whenever he leaves the facility). You may also request copies of medication administration reports if you wish, but this is not usually necessary. Be sure to keep copies of all the records you send to the new facility.

- Inform hospice or nursing agencies caring for your loved one about the change. If equipment needs to be moved, such as a hospital bed or an oxygen concentrator, contact the company that owns it. They will usually want to move it themselves. They probably will issue new equipment and pick up the old one after the move.

- Upon arriving at the new facility, introduce Mom to the staff and a few residents who may be out and about. If she's up to it, give her a little tour of her new home. Otherwise, show her to her room and let her lie down for a rest, saving the tour for when she has more energy. Try to highlight things about the home that you know she will appreciate. Once Mom is settled, give copies of the above reports to the manager. Find out who is the best person to talk to about her needs, likes and dislikes. You can waste a lot of time telling the owners that Mom hates mayonnaise but really loves her 3:00 gin and tonic, when they are not going to be the ones making her sandwich or planning out happy hour. Talk to the manager or the key caregivers who will be caring for her. It is always appropriate to ask, "Who should I talk to about Mom's preferences?" Communicate what was unsatisfactory at the former place so that you do not experience the same thing in the new place.

WHEN YOUR LOVED ONE PASSES AWAY

A little planning can make this time of loss for family and friends a lot more peaceful for everyone. Death is a reality for everybody, and plans that were made earlier, while you were all in your right minds, allows you to focus on your own grieving and the needs of family and friends.

Usually the facility will charge for as many days as the resident's things are left in the room. It is a good idea to designate someone to move Dad's personal belongings out promptly. You will be very busy and everyone will be grieving, and you can spend several hundred dollars unnecessarily by waiting a week to clear out the room.

The facility is obligated to refund any unused fees for the remainder of the month after the room is vacated. They have thirty days to refund your fees, petty cash, and deposit money.

CHAPTER 6

Oh No! I Didn't Plan!

YOU'RE NOT ALONE

Yes, we know you're out there—we see you every day. Even if you haven't planned ahead, all the tips and information in this book will be helpful, and we highly recommend reading it cover to cover. That's why we made it short.

Most of the important things you need to know are here. However, we have included a special section for you so that you can have a step-by-step guide to some critical things to know in order to avoid major pitfalls.

STEP 1

If you need to place your loved one quickly, start by going to our website at www.arizonahomestead.com. There you can fill out a brief questionnaire and someone will contact you within twenty-four hours to discuss your needs and be your personal advisor.

STEP 2

Obtain a TB skin test for your loved one. You will need this anywhere you go, and it takes at least forty-eight hours to read.

STEP 3

If possible, discuss with Mom and Dad what is most important to them. Some things that might lead you to a smaller home are personal care needs (toileting, transferring, fall risk), fully prepared meals, services like laundry and housekeeping, and medication management. If these are real needs, the smaller home is much better equipped to carry them out at a much higher standard, as they will almost always have a better ratio of staff to residents. A larger facility would cater better to a more independent individual who may need limited physical assistance but wants a larger social community and transportation to shopping and doctor visits. Because of the staff to resident ratio in larger facilities, residents will wait longer for assistance and are largely left on their own for socialization or participation in activities. If Mom or Dad require more complex medical care, you may need to consider a skilled nursing facility.

STEP 4

Determine how much the family is willing to spend. This will help tremendously in your search for a home. Remember that the costs are very real for the care institution, and you will most likely get only what you pay for and little more. If money is an issue, decide how the family can contribute to enhance what the facility is able to provide.

STEP 5

If your time is short, you may benefit greatly from contacting a referral agent. The facility releasing your family member will most likely give you the name of someone who can help. You can also go to our website at www.arizonahomestead.com and we will do our best to help you find a facility that meets your needs.

The Arizona Department of Health Services Assisted Living website lists the names and locations of homes with their zip codes, and they also list the most recent inspection reports online. You may want to check this site to make sure you aren't overlooking a good option nearby that may not be contracted with your referral agent.

A Final Word of Encouragement

Making the transition into a long-term care environment always involves a certain amount of anxiety, uncertainty, and stress. There will be a sense of loss of freedom and the end of life as you knew it. We hope we have given you a sense of how the system works so that the transition is a bit smoother.

It will help you to know you aren't alone and that there are resources in the community for you. Our suggestion is that you and your family enter into this transition with an open heart. Welcome opportunities for growth, and look for new relationships that might even turn into lifelong friendships. Keep a positive attitude and find reasons to be grateful. Look for ways you can bring happiness to your loved one and to others in her new community. Only you can determine what you bring to the experience, and we hope that you will bring hope and optimism with you to your relative's new home.

Appendix 1

EVALUATING CARE-HOME QUALITY AND SUITABILITY

This is one of the trickiest things you will ever do for your loved one. Keep in mind that one of the best indicators of a good home is how you feel as you walk through the facility. Even if you cannot pinpoint why you feel good or bad about a place, take those feelings seriously. A bad feeling may be as simple as a personality conflict, but the high level of trust you must place in those caring for Mom or Dad will come a lot easier if your overall feeling is positive.

Here are some questions to ask the administration and staff. Questions to ask yourself as you tour are shown in parentheses. Note the details you feel are most important before you begin looking for a facility.

- What levels of care do you provide? Are there adequate safeguards in place for directed care? Are there secure outdoor areas for unattended residents? Is the staff equipped for your loved one's specific needs?
- What is the staffing ratio? Is that guaranteed? (At first glance, do the caregivers look like people with whom Mom will feel comfortable? Are they clean and dressed neatly? Are they alert and attentive?)
- (Do the residents look clean, cared for, happy? At first glance, do you think Mom will get along with them?) How are wandering residents handled?
- What are the costs? What does that include? What are the added charges?

- Does the facility have nurse practitioners or doctors who visit the home? How often? What is their role in patient care? How do they get paid? How are prescriptions handled?
- Is there a security deposit? Is it refundable? Is there a community fee?
- Do you provide transportation? If so, who drives and in what vehicle?
- Are electric wheelchairs allowed? What are the restrictions? Do they pose a hazard to mobility?
- What activities do you provide? Do people come in for special activities? Do you provide for spiritual needs? How are activities tailored to the needs and interests of the residents?
- Can residents choose between eating in their rooms or going to the dining room? How are food preferences and special diets handled? Is there an extra charge? (Does the food look appetizing? Are the meals healthful?)
- What are the alcohol, smoking, and pet policies? (Are you comfortable with them? How do you feel about pets on the premises?)
- (What does the home smell like? Does it look and feel clean? Is the lighting adequate? Is the temperature comfortable for you? Do you think it will be comfortable for your family member?)
- (Is there a positive attitude in the home? Are residents out and about? People might be napping at mid-morning and mid-afternoon, so there would be less activity at those times. Observe the facility at different times of day.)
- Is it all right if I drop in unannounced and roam around?

Appendix 2

Quality-of-Life Care Plan

Name

_____

Likes to be called

_____

Favorite Foods

_____
_____

Food Dislikes

_____
_____

Activity Preferences

_____
_____
_____

Brief History of Life and Accomplishments

_____
_____
_____

Quality of Life Factors: (Please list those things we can do to maximize the resident's quality of life.)

_____
_____
_____
_____

Acknowledgments

We would like to acknowledge those who have made the writing of this book possible. First, I thank God for the incredible opportunity He has given us to work in this industry and to participate in the lives of so many people at such a profound time. We have been so blessed and enriched as a result. I also thank Him for the strength to make it through the rough times—and there have been many—and for the subsequent growth and maturity He has brought about in our own lives as a result. It has been through the development of our own business that we have gained the education and knowledge to produce this book.

We would also like to thank our kids, Samuel, Jonathan, and Katie, for their incredible ability not only to hang in there and become amazing young adults, but also for the contributions of hard work, ideas, and moral support that they have given over the years. We could not have built this business without their help, patience, and understanding on so many occasions.

Next we must thank the Arizona Homestead residents, staff, and families who have educated us from the beginning. We started with very little knowledge of either long-term care or business, but have learned on the way and have appreciated those who have been there and given us the opportunity to serve them while at the same time learning, sometimes by trial and error.

Finally, we would like to say thank you to the Arizona Dept. of Health Services for its support of those caring for our seniors. We truly feel that, in being there for our residents, you are there for us and our success as we work as a team to provide the highest possible quality of life for those in our community.

Index

www.ingramcontent.com/pod-product-compliance
Lightning Source LLC
Chambersburg PA
CBHW021246280526
45784CB00005B/2256